# MASSAGE
# The Art of Massage Aiding in Diabetes, Backache, Anxiety, Depression and Much More

BRENDA HERRERA

ISBN: 9781981076086

# DEDICATION


This book has a special dedication to God, my family, students, co-workers, and a very special person in my life. You have all left a footprint in my heart.

# CONTENTS

# DISCLAIMER

This book has been written to provide information on the benefit of massage in diabetes and other conditions. Every effort has been made to make this information as complete and accurate as possible.
Also, this book contains information on the benefit of massage in diabetes and other conditions, only up to the publishing date. Therefore, this report should be used as a guide – not as the ultimate source of information on the topic.

The purpose of this book is to educate. The author does not warrant that the information contained in this book is fully complete and shall not be responsible for any errors or omissions.

The author shall have neither liability nor responsibility to any person or entity with respect to any loss or damage caused or alleged to be caused directly or indirectly by this book.

# INTRODUCTION

Massage therapy has been in practice for centuries with references apparent in prehistoric writings from dynasties including Egypt, Mesopotamia, China, Japan, and India. This therapy involves the art of muscle and soft tissue manipulation manually in order to provide physical and mental relief. There are over 80 different massaging styles in practice at present. Each technique utilizes a specific set of movements over different pressure points. Gentle stroking, kneading, rubbing, pressing, tapping, and vibration are namely some of the numerous motions used in this ancient therapy. The styles used in massage therapy span over long smooth stroking motions to short more percussive ones.

Essential oils and ointments are often used in conjunction with massaging thereby incorporating aromatherapy into the art form. Massage therapy aims at not only physical relief but also mental relaxation. Stress control is an integral outcome of massage therapy along with other benefits that go beyond the realm of simply peace of mind and body. So what exactly are the benefits of massage therapy? Here is a list of health conditions that can be effectively healed and aided through massage therapy.

### Backache

Various studies have proved the correlation between massage therapy and backache relief. Many even consider it to be more effective than spinal modification or acupuncture. Massaging has reduced the need for prescription painkillers by approximately a staggering 40%.

### Headache

Studies have revealed that massage therapy is capable of reducing the incidence of migraines in an individual and also is said to aid in overall improved sleep patterns.

### Anxiety and Depression

Mental illness, unfortunately, is an often overlooked aspect of general wellbeing. With occurrences of anxiety and depression on the rise, a relationship between the physiological workings of the human body and psychological behaviors has been established.

The Art of Massage Aiding in Diabetes, Backache, Anxiety, Depression and Much More

**Anxiety and depression are the results of increased cortisol hormone levels in the body.**

Massage therapy actively reduces the cortisol level in the body by a staggering 50%. Furthermore, the movements utilized in this therapy have been proven to increase neurotransmitter release in the body that aids in alleviating depression.

## Cancer

Cancer is a very commonly encountered disease that is only deemed curable through intensive treatments using Western medicine. While it may seem that massage therapy has no role to play on the road to recovery, it plays an integral role in dealing with the psychological aspects of the illness. Having to deal with a terminal illness is already stressful for the body to deal with. The psychological aspect of the treatment process involves depression, nausea, fatigue, chronic pain and compromised immunity. To help reduce the above-mentioned side effects of cancer treatment, massage therapy has managed to be extremely effective. Many Clients who sought massage therapy in conjunction with regular chemotherapy and radiotherapy also exhibited a better response to the treatment with their recovery journey being overall more positive than others.

## Arthritis

Bone Degenerative Diseases are on the rise largely due to unhealthy eating habits, genetic factors, and general sedentary lifestyle choices. Massage therapy has come to the help of those suffering from osteoarthritis by resulting in reduced pain and stiffness and improved joint function.

**Now that we are well aware of the benefits of massage therapy, let's move on to its relationship with diabetes.**

# CHAPTER 1

# UNDERSTANDING TYPE 2 DIABETES

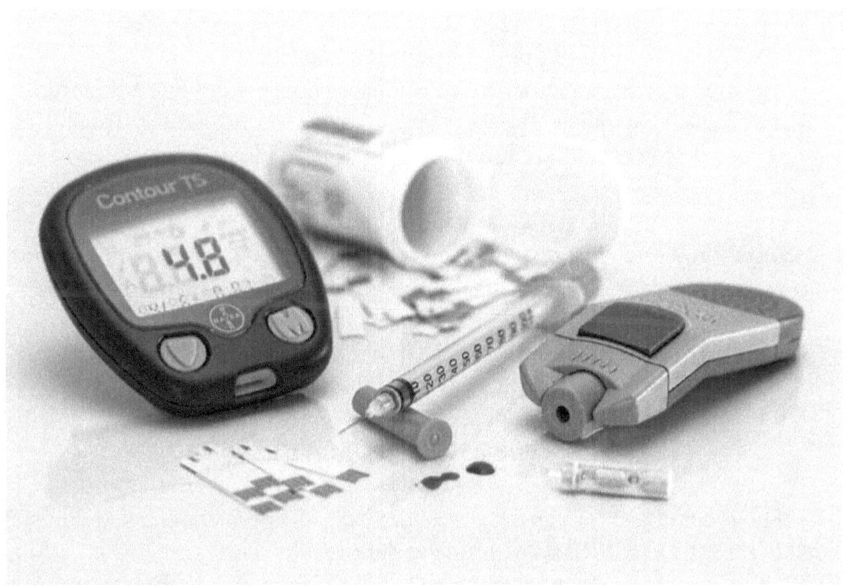

Source: Pexels

## What exactly is Type 2 Diabetes?

Diabetes Type 2 is essentially the resultant condition after the pancreas fails to produce the hormone insulin or when the human body refuses to accept insulin. Insulin is the hormone that is responsible for blood sugar regulation by metabolizing carbohydrates. Due to the lack of insulin in the body's circulation, impaired carbohydrate metabolism results in the resting blood sugar levels remain elevated. A persistently elevated level of glucose in the blood is referred to as Diabetes Mellitus.

Diabetes Mellitus is a broad term that encompasses various systemic symptoms and signs. This disease is categorized into different types; each resulting from specific causative factors.

### Type 1 Diabetes Mellitus

Also often referred to as Juvenile Diabetes, Type 1 Diabetes Mellitus is often found in young individuals such as children and young adults. This category of Diabetes Mellitus results due to the autoimmune destruction of pancreatic beta cells; that is responsible for the production of insulin. The onset of this condition has been notified to be caused by physical or emotional stress. Type 1 Diabetes Mellitus results in low production of insulin due to the pancreatic impairment, therefore, all Type 1 Diabetes Mellitus Clients must be given insulin injections in order to survive. The prevalence of this variant ranges from 10-15% of the diabetic population.

### Type 1.5 Diabetes Mellitus

An intermediate category that exhibits symptoms that are evident in both Type 1 as well as Type 2, Type 1.5 Diabetes Mellitus is usually encountered in middle-aged individuals.

### Gestational Diabetes

Gestational Diabetes results when the fetus impairs the mother's ability to respond appropriately to insulin thereby resulting in increased blood sugar.

The most common variant prevalent in a huge percentage of the general population, however, is Type 2 Diabetes Mellitus.

### Type 2 Diabetes Mellitus

The most common variant of the disease is Type 2 Diabetes Mellitus. Unlike Type 1 Diabetes Mellitus, this variant results when one of two things happens. One, when the pancreatic cells fail to produce a sufficient amount of insulin that is required to maintain normal blood glucose levels. Two, when the body becomes incapable of utilizing the insulin that is being produced by the pancreas. Regardless of the underlying reason, the end result involves elevated blood glucose levels. Affecting more than 85% of diabetics, this disease requires oral medication that aims at lowering the body's resistance to insulin and subsequently enhances its sensitivity response. In advanced cases, the clients may require insulin injections for blood glucose level maintenance.

The Art of Massage Aiding in Diabetes, Backache, Anxiety, Depression and Much More

Now that we have discussed the basics of this condition, let's dive into the specifics of this condition such as the signs, symptoms, and prescribed treatments necessary to control the disease.

## Causes

Diabetes Mellitus can result from a wide array of causative factors. The most common ones include obesity and inactive lifestyle choices. Other factors include trauma, genetics, glandular dysfunction, etc.

## Signs and Symptoms

Like any other disease, diabetes comes with its own set of evident symptoms and signs that lead to an accurate diagnosis. The most common symptoms include excessive urination; excessive thirst; lethargy; paresthesia, or tingling or burning sensation; neuropathy, and weight problems. Fatigue results largely due to the cells being deprived of energy. Due to glucose and sugars being wasted with urine, the body's cells crave more water. This need to compensate for hydration presents itself in the form of excessive thirst and thus, frequent episodes of urination.

## Complications

The most commonly encountered complications associated with Diabetes Mellitus comprise of cardiovascular disease, dental disease, kidney disease, amputations, impaired vision, and neuromuscular disorders such as neuropathy. Other changes may involve the soft tissue and connective tissue in the body in the form of thickened or stiff fascia that surrounds other organs, bones, muscles, etc.

## Treatment

Diabetes Mellitus cannot be cured. However, it can be controlled. Diabetes Mellitus treatment lays primary focus towards the maintenance and normalization of blood glucose levels in the body. A healthy person's normal resting blood glucose ranges from 80 to 120 mg/dl. The goal of diabetes treatment is to maintain a healthy balance between medication, physical exercise, adequate nutrition, and stress management. This balance maintenance requires careful monitoring. The fastest and most convenient method of keeping blood glucose levels in check is by employing strip tests. On accounts of fluctuations in blood glucose levels, adequate measures can be taken in order to keep a client healthy. Monitoring also helps in deducing any need for dosage adjustment. Common medications employed to control diabetes include the following:

- **Pig pancreatic transplantation:** Replacing the affected organ with Pig insulin as it is almost the best-match to human insulin.
- **Sulfonylureas:** Stimulates the release of insulin from the pancreas.
- **Metformin:** Reduces the amount of glucose released from the liver.
- **Starlix and Prandin:** Both trigger insulin release from the pancreas
- **Alpha-Glucosidase Inhibitors:** Slows down the digestion of carbs.
- **DPP-4 Inhibitors:** Lower blood sugar levels.

Diabetes is not an illness that will cripple you or deprive you of enjoying all different aspects of life. All you need is a balance. With proper medical treatment and actively invoking healthy lifestyle choices into one's everyday routine, diabetics are capable of leading perfectly normal lives.

**So what is exactly the correlation between massage therapy and diabetes management? First, let's take a closer look at the basic issues of a diabetic person that can be tackled by massage therapy.**

# CHAPTER 2

# CIRCULATION AND NEUROPATHY ISSUES IN DIABETES

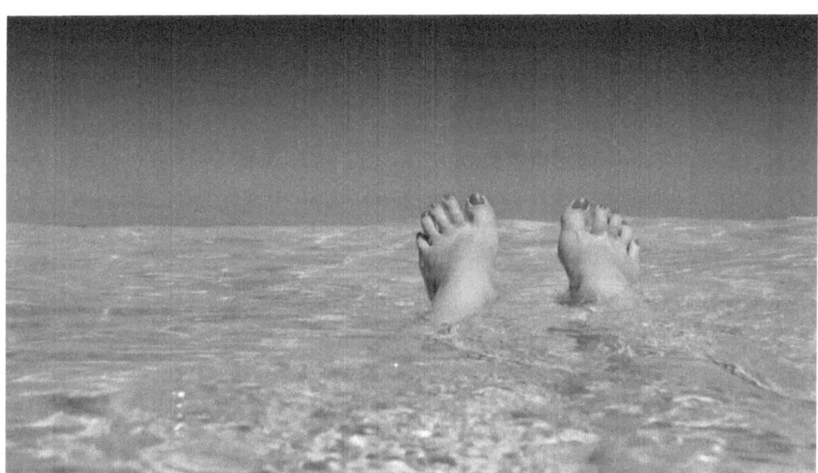

Source: Pexels

**Effects of diabetes on blood circulation**

With millions of people across the globe suffering from diabetes mellitus, a common side effect observed include poor circulation of blood. Increased blood glucose levels result in a number of circulatory problems around the body with common examples being increased disability and complications that can potentially affect your life. These problems can potentially worsen if a good control isn't kept on the body's sugar level.

**Types of circulatory problems in diabetic clients:**

The following types of circulatory problems are commonly seen in Clients suffering from diabetes mellitus.

1. **Peripheral artery disease**- this side effect results in diminished blood flow to the peripheries of the legs and feet. When performing activities such as walking, not enough blood flow reaches those areas, a condition commonly known as intermittent claudication.
2. **Diabetic retinopathy**- when decreased blood reaches the small blood vessels of the eyes, they become damaged. This means diabetic retinopathy can potentially result in complete blindness or partial vision loss.
3. **Kidney damage**- insufficient supply of blood to the renal vessels will eventually lead to damage to the kidneys.

**Symptoms commonly observed in diabetics due to poor circulatory problems:**

There are a number of symptoms that can be associated with poor circulation due to diabetes. This includes the following:

- Chest pain during activities that cause exertion
- Pain in the extremities such as the legs and feet while walking
- Increased levels of blood pressure
- A rise in the incidence of foot infections due to diminished blood flow
- Difficulty in seeing, partial vision loss
- Fatigue, retention of fluids and observance of proteins in the urine
- Breakdown of skin, especially in the foot region

**Effects of massage on the problems associated with poor circulatory problems in diabetics**

- Helps to promote blood flow into a particular region that is deprived of blood. This means all the problems mentioned above such as renal damage, retinal damage and periphery damage can all be reduced greatly.
- Removes or flushes out the stored buildup of lactic acid from the body's muscles. This helps to remove fatigue associated with performing everyday normal activities.
- Allows the delivery of fresh, oxygen-rich blood into the body, energizing the body like before. All activities that the body was not

able to perform can now easily be done.

- Eases soreness of muscle that arises due to blood congestion
- Enhanced mobility due to increased blood circulation of the legs and feet

Understanding diabetic neuropathy

Diabetic neuropathy is the name given to damage to your nerves as a result of increased blood glucose levels in the blood for a long duration.

## Common types of neuropathy that affect diabetics

- Peripheral Neuropathy- a type of neuropathy affecting the peripheries of the hands and feet
- Autonomic Neuropathy- a type of neuropathy that affects the digestive tract primarily. Blood vessels, sex organs, and the urinary tract may also be affected.

## Common symptoms of neuropathy in diabetic individuals

### 1. Peripheral neuropathy

- Numbness which may become permanent after a while
- Tingling sensations
- Painful sensations
- Feeling of burns, especially during the evening time

### 2. Autonomic neuropathy

- Frequent spells of diarrhea
- Feeling of bloating
- Constant urge of vomiting
- Nausea feeling frequently observed
- Eating small meals and feeling extremely full
- Sensations of heartburn throughout the day
- Constipation frequently observed

## Effects of massage on the problems related to diabetic neuropathy

Massages have been observed to bring about a vast improvement in those suffering from diabetes mellitus. This includes the following:
- Releases endorphins, body's natural painkillers
- Aids in the reduction of spasms and cramping
- Helps to alleviate nerve pain and paresthesia that occurs frequently
- Improves circulation by pumping essential nutrients into the body
- Improves bowel habits and reduces constipation/bloating

# CHAPTER 3

# BLOOD GLUCOSE AWARENESS –THE BASIC CONCERN OF DIABETIC PERSON

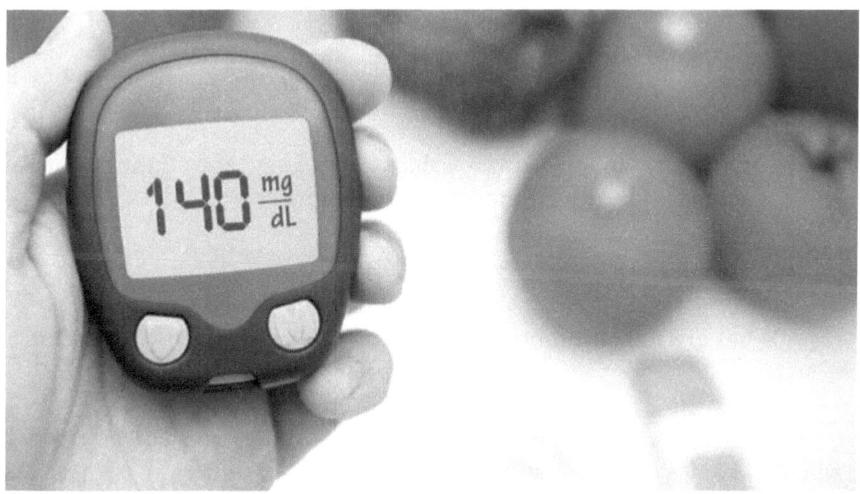

Source: Pinterest

With diabetes mellitus being so prevalent in the world's population, it should come as no surprise that blood glucose awareness should be a matter stressed and promoted amongst us all. Learning about how to sense a drop or rise in sugar levels, common symptoms of hypoglycemia, how to manage such situations and how you can prevent them is crucial for the wellbeing of diabetic individuals. It is important to remember that in diabetic individuals, severe hypoglycemia is considered to be a medical emergency that requires careful attention to be treated. Let's take a look at the following ways you can become more blood glucose aware.

## What are the common symptoms associated with low blood glucose levels?

Hypoglycemia or low blood sugar levels are a frequently observed condition in all diabetics, especially those who have been diagnosed with Type 1 diabetes. The following symptoms are commonly seen in such Clients:

- Perspiration
- Mouth tingling
- Fingers trembling
- Increased heart rate
- Shaking
- Trembling all over the body
- Weakness
- Feeling of being unwell or malaise
- Dizziness
- Vague or confused feeling
- Sleepiness
- Difficulty in speaking, walking, thinking and during normal activities like driving and operating machinery
- Loss of consciousness and coma
- Convulsions/ fits/ seizures

## What are the common risk factors associated with the cause of hypoglycemia?

Hypoglycemia as mentioned previously is a major medical emergency when it comes to those involved in diabetes. In order to help create awareness and prevent this condition, it's necessary to know about the common risk factors involved. This includes the following:

1. **Missing or delaying a regular meal-** it's no surprise that food means calories and nutrients. When your body misses or delays a meal, the level of glucose in the blood decreases to a great extent. This means you no longer have the energy to carry out your normal activities. Diabetic individuals already have decreased levels of glucose storage so that means depriving the body of its main nutrient can result in disastrous consequences.

The Art of Massage Aiding in Diabetes, Backache, Anxiety, Depression and Much More

2. **Ingesting an overdose of a certain medication-** there are a number of medications that can cause drops in your blood glucose levels, insulin being a common one for diabetics with type 1 diabetes.
3. **Alcohol consumption-** alcohol is known to cause blood sugar levels to fall to a drastic low. It does this by preventing the body's liver from releasing glycogen into the bloodstream. Glycogen is necessary for the proper functioning and maintenance of glucose levels.
4. **Indulging in forms of strenuous exercise-** it's a known fact that exercise of any form or type requires energy in the form of glucose. Taking part in exercise causes depletion of stored glycogen reserves and for this reason, hypoglycemia can commonly be observed in such individuals.

### How to treat hypoglycemia conditions effectively?

The level and extent of treatment for hypoglycemia totally depend on how conscious the person involved is.

- If an individual is suffering from an emergency situation of severe hypoglycemia, administration of glucagon via a glucagon injection kit is necessary. This is considered as one of the safest and most effective ways of raising blood glucose levels. It is, however, important to ensure that the client who is getting the respective glucagon administration is in the position of recovery. This is done in an effort to prevent a case of vomiting that may follow glucagon administration.
- If the individual involved is conscious and glucagon isn't available immediately, a sweet such as a candy, fruit, chocolate or fruit juice can be administered in an attempt to raise the blood glucose levels.
- In situations where the Client is semi-conscious or unconscious, feeding items should be avoided at all costs in an attempt to prevent choking. With that being said, glucagon may be attempted to be given I/V in a clinical setup by a medical professional.

### How to ensure that your blood glucose levels are in check and balance?

Being a known diabetic, it's crucial to always keep your glucose levels in check and balance at all times. This is done in an effort to ensure that everything stays close to normal limits. Diabetes, as mentioned previously, is known to affect the body's entire mechanism. High blood glucose levels result in damage to vital organs such as the eyes and kidney. Other than that, it imbalances the hormonal mechanism in such a way that circulation of blood is drastically affected. The following ways are great for keeping your blood glucose levels in total check and balance at all times.

### Know your blood sugar levels.

This includes the normal range and how much you can exceed within those limits.

### Visit your endocrinologist every 3 months for consultation.
Discuss any matters or issues you may be having.

### Keep a check on your legs and feet.

High blood glucose levels are known to affect the extremities to a severe extent. This is done in an effort to reduce deranged mobility, neuropathy and other common symptoms. This means regular visits to the dermatologist and suggestions for proper foot care.

### Eat a balanced diet full of nutrients.

This will allow your body to get the desired calories to carry out everyday activities.

### Avoid unnecessary sweets
They can further aggravate high blood glucose levels, leading to further damage. Perform regular glucose testing so as to be aware of the direction in which your body is heading in terms of sugar.

### Never skip or delay meals.
This will only further harm your body in an irreversible manner.

### Exercise daily
Weight gain can again decrease your body's sensitivity to the effects of insulin.

### Follow the Treatment Regime

The Art of Massage Aiding in Diabetes, Backache, Anxiety, Depression and Much More

If you're a type 1 diabetic individual, you must follow your prescribed treatment regimen of insulin intake. Those who are type 2 diabetics; they are obliged to follow the treatment regimen of oral hypoglycemic drugs as prescribed by the doctor. Any change in dosages should be discussed by a medical doctor and not done based on one's personal judgment. Knowing the symptoms of hypoglycemia is necessary as this is an emergency that can possibly occur at any point in time of a diabetic individual's life.

**Blood sugar awareness when it comes to Massage Therapy**

It is recommended by health professionals around the globe that diabetic individuals take precautions in an attempt of avoiding hypoglycemia during a massage treatment. Precautions should never be overlooked when involved in any activity. During a massage, however, extra care is required. This is because massage therapy is a form of treatment where restful relaxation makes it easier to overlook the symptoms related to an insulin reaction.

Before the treatment begins, it's important for the client to inform the massage therapist of the possibility of hypoglycemia and how the client manages to deal with it. Blood sugar levels should be checked after leaving the massage session so as to ensure that the calming effects of the massage can be enjoyed.

# CHAPTER 4

# MYOFASCIAL EFFECTS

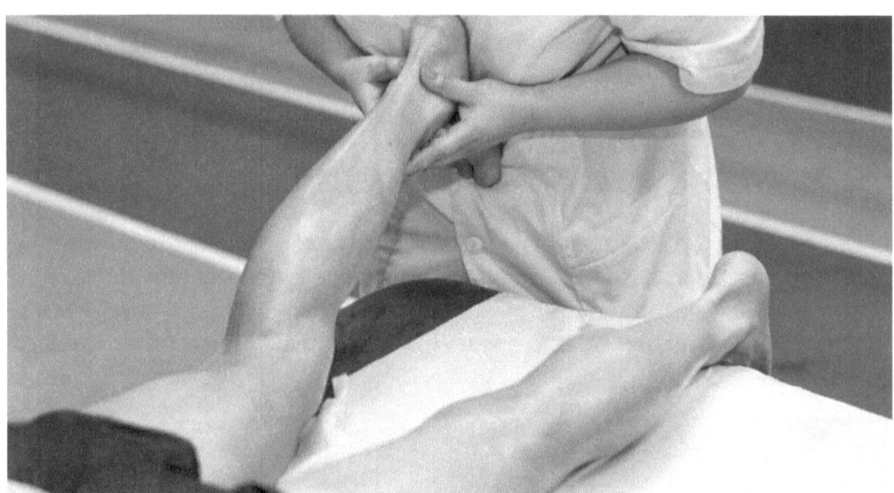

SOURCE: ENDOSTOCK

Diabetes mellitus is known for affecting the musculoskeletal system in a number of ways. The effects are known to take a toll on the entire body. Increased blood sugar levels thicken the connective tissue linings of the skin and fascia. This means deranged mobility and pain on movement can result. Other than that, a whole series of myofascial effects are commonly seen in these types of Clients. This includes the following:

- Neuropathic joints
- Muscle cramps

- Stiff Hands Syndrome
- Carpal Tunnel Syndrome
- Tenosynovitis
- Limited joint mobility
- Peripheral Neuropathy
- Muscle Infarction
- Diffuse Idiopathic Skeletal Hyperostosis
- Adhesive capsulitis of the shoulder

## Neuropathic joints

This condition is known to cause severe joint destruction, most commonly involving the feet region. It may also lead to loss of sensory innervations and difficulty in mobility.

## Muscle cramps and infarction

Muscle cramps and infarction commonly result due to a diminished supply of blood in the body. It's a potentially disabling condition that occurs on a spontaneous basis. This condition is more commonly seen in those Clients diagnosed with diabetes mellitus type 1. Ischemia or reduced blood flow causes damage to the micro vessels and this further aggravates the condition into one of infarction. The most commonly affected region involved is said to be the lower leg and calf region. Normal activities generally don't aggravate the condition. However, extreme forms of exercise can be deleterious.

## Stiff hands syndrome

The hand region is a common target in diabetic Clients for a number of reasons. The skin of the hands becomes tight, thick and waxy in texture. There are a number of factors associated with this condition. This includes an increased breakdown of collagen, increased levels of glycosylation of the skin's collagen and diabetic neuropathy too. In advanced stages of this condition, the fingers can undergo flexion contracture. One common indication of stiff hands syndrome is that Client will be unable to press the palms of his hands together. As a result of this, a gap will ultimately remain when the palms and fingers are pressed together.

## Limited joint mobility

When the joints are covered by excess thickening of the fascia and connective tissue linings, limited joint mobility ultimately results. This means difficulty in movements, pain on movements and extreme debilitation into one's life.

## Carpal Tunnel Syndrome

Carpal tunnel syndrome is the name given to a condition commonly associated with diabetic Clients. In this condition, entrapment of the median nerve results due to a prolonged increase in blood glucose levels as well as the degenerative connective tissue changes that result due to diabetes mellitus. In this condition, the Client will generally complain of sensory loss, paresthesia, and burning sensations around the area where the median nerve is located. Pain may also radiate towards the region of the elbow and forearm. Clients in this condition fight it extremely difficult and painful to undergo simple everyday movements like flexion, extension and other wrist movements.

## Adhesive capsulitis of the shoulder region

Another myofascial side effect that occurs due to abnormal glucose levels in diabetic individuals is stiffness and limited movement of the glenohumeral shoulder joint. Thickening of the shoulder capsule occurs commonly and this ultimately results in contracture of the shoulder's joint capsule. Simple shoulder movements such as abduction, external and internal rotation are carried out with great pain and difficulty.

## Tenosynovitis

This condition may also be referred to as trigger finger. It affects the hands of a diabetic individual where clients may complain of their fingers becoming tightened or locked with a sensation of discomfort. Nodules that are palpable are a distinct clinical finding observed in most affected Clients. Active or passive flexion of the fingers may also reproduce the symptoms of tenosynovitis.

## Diffuse skeletal hyperostosis

The condition of diffuse skeletal hyperostosis is one where the paraspinal ligaments undergo calcification. It is more commonly observed

The Art of Massage Aiding in Diabetes, Backache, Anxiety, Depression and Much More

in those Clients with diabetes mellitus type 2 where obesity is the most common risk factor for these clients. In diffuse skeletal hyperostosis, clients will generally complain of symptoms relating to neck stiffness, back stiffness, and decreased the range of movements. The most common sites of the human body involved include the thoracic region, the spine in particular. Other than that, the cervical spine and lumbar regions are involved.

## How can an individual with diabetes mellitus prevent or reduce the incidence of these myofascial effects?

If you want to bring about a reduction in the incidence of the following features being mentioned above, maintaining normal blood sugar levels is the first step to success. This means keeping track of previous blood sugar levels and comparing them with current ones. Improvement should be the key focus and methods derived to bring about that improvement should be part of your everyday treatment regimen. Only when you have a command on your body's glycemic index, secondary preventive measures such as physiotherapy, steroid injections, and analgesics can be sought as medical forms of therapy from your respected doctor.

## Can massage therapy be sought as a therapy for the reduction of myofascial effects in diabetic individuals?

The answer to this question is a simple yes. Myofascial effects can be relieved through the therapy of a massage. It's all about delivering the right type and form of movements to the affected region and the results of doing so through massage therapy are miraculous. The following results can be observed after a massage therapy:

- Increased tissue elasticity
- Greater extent of mobility
- Greater levels of flexibility
- Reduction in stiffness and pain around the joint region
- Greater delivery of oxygen and blood to the periphery areas
- Improved strength and texture of the muscles and fascia region
- Reduction in the fascia lining that surrounds the vital organs and muscles

Now that we have taken a deep insight into the issues related to diabetes, let's take a look at what are the benefits of aiding massage therapy into diabetes treatment.

# 5 POSSIBLE ADVANTAGES OF MASSAGE THERAPY IN DIABETES

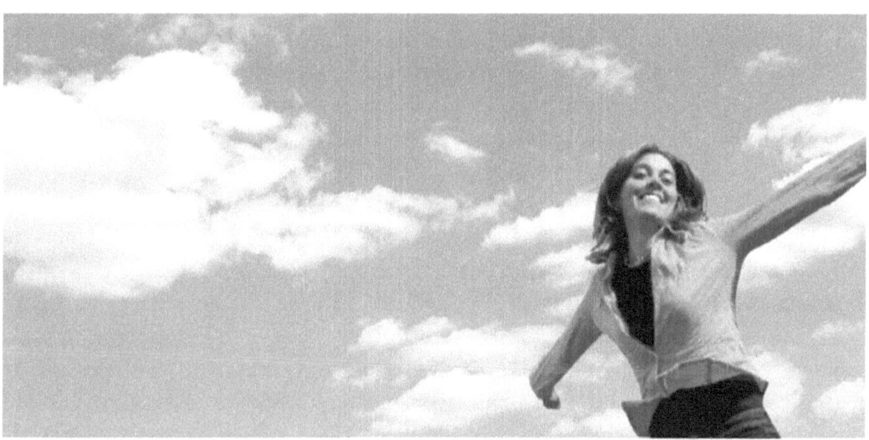

When it comes to diabetes mellitus, there are a number of complications that may arise due to this ailment. To help bring about an improvement in the effects of diabetes, massage therapy has been seen as a wonderful treatment modality for aiding diabetes. Be it type 1 or type 2 diabetes, diabetics can greatly benefit from professional massage therapy. Being diabetic means welcoming a whole lot of stress into one's life.

Dealing with stress means allowing the human body to respond in such a way that blood glucose levels are raised. This is known as the fight or flight response, instilled in every individual. From lowering blood pressure and heart rate to muscle relaxation and increased endorphin release, the benefits of massage therapy to be gained by individuals suffering from diabetes are immense. Let's take a closer look at these benefits in detail.

## Increased blood circulation regulation

Increased blood glucose levels can lead to poor circulation of blood throughout the body. With that being said, massages are a great form of therapy that aid in improving and promoting circulation throughout the human body. There are a number of distinct massages that hold this benefit and they include the following:

- Regular massage
- Deep muscle therapy
- Relaxation massage
- Hot stone envy

The following forms of massage therapy being mentioned above are known to greatly improve blood flow in one particular area such as those where congestion has occurred. This allows lactic acid to be flushed from your body's muscles, enabling oxygen-rich blood to reach all the deprived areas. Special note: Make sure the diabetes is controlled. If the diabetes is not controlled avoid the massage and get a medical release.

## Diminishing the effects of neuropathy

Neuropathy is a known complication of diabetes that affects a great majority of the world's population. Neuropathy can be associated with pain or more commonly with loss of sensation. Massage therapy can greatly improve neuropathy by helping to raise the levels of endorphins released by the body into the bloodstream. Increased endorphins release results in raising the body's threshold for pain. Massage therapies such as Sports Massage and Trigger Point Therapy are two great therapies for releasing endorphins like oxytocin and serotonin. Both these endorphins are great for relieving suffering from chronic pain. Neuropathy associated with loss of sensation can also be treated with great ease using massage and reflexology techniques. Restoration of nerve function as well as sensation are two added benefits brought about through the use of massage. This allows the client to help stay on a proper treatment regimen.

## Friction and scar removal

In diabetes mellitus, getting frequent insulin injections is a common form of treatment for those suffering from type 1 or insulin-dependent diabetes. It is very common to observe nerve injury that further leads to scar development in these types of Clients. When taking on massage and

The Art of Massage Aiding in Diabetes, Backache, Anxiety, Depression and Much More

reflexology techniques, pain and dysfunction can greatly be reduced at chronic injection sites. Usually, in these types of Clients, excess buildup of scar tissue causes the skin to thicken, drastically affecting mobility. Massage therapy is a wonderful way to remove friction and scars, helping to restore mobility in debilitated diabetic clients.

## Ultimate form of relaxation and soothing

As mentioned previously, diabetes mellitus brings with it a baggage of stress to whoever may be suffering from it. To help cope with all that stress, massages are an excellent form of therapy that provides a soothing and relaxation filled experience. The mechanism of action through which all this occurs is simple. Sedation of the body's nervous system allows diabetic individuals to attain the rest and wellbeing of the body that is required. It is a known fact that stress has the ability to take a toll on the entire body. To help restore a diabetic individual's hormonal organic balance, calming the nervous system is crucial. What better way of doing so than by easing the mind and body through a massage.

## Positive myofascial effects

Increased blood glucose levels such as that in diabetes are famous for causing thickening of the body's connective tissue lining. These results in loss of elasticity and mobility of the body. Stiff tendons, muscles, and ligaments are a norm as well as joints depicting a decreased range of movement. Diabetic individuals no longer have to feel restricted to living a sedentary lifestyle. This is because another great advantage of getting massages are the numerous myofascial benefits that come with its usage.

The benefits include greater tissue elasticity as well as more effective mobility. Depression can be cured thoroughly as clients can get relief from restricted movement and mood swings related to depression. This a great form of psychological boost to diabetes sufferers.

When it comes to diabetes, motivation to carry on with a healthy and stress-free lifestyle can be difficult for many out there. Massages are great for giving that extra bit of boost psychologically to those living on the edge of a breakdown. The sheer motivation one gets from a massage can make an individual strive to attain all the necessary factors needed to live a healthy and balanced lifestyle, despite having diabetes.

**So, how do we incorporate the benefits of massage therapy as an aid to diabetes treatment? Read on to know the secret.**

# CHAPTER 6

## SAFE PRESSURE POINT MASSAGE TECHNIQUES FOR DIABETIC INDIVIDUALS

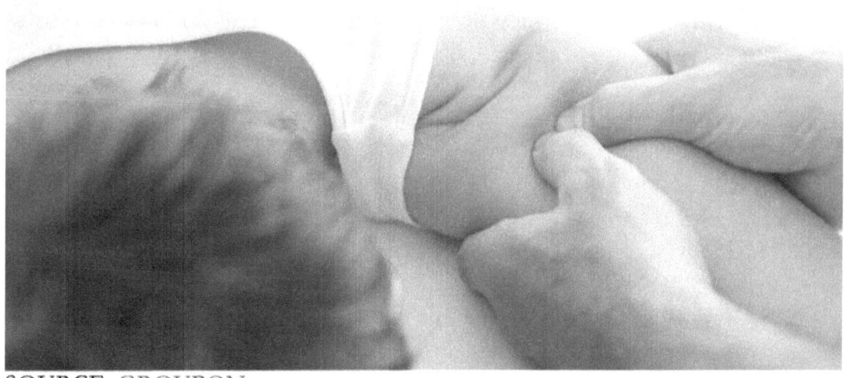

SOURCE: GROUPON

With diabetes being one of the most common medical conditions affecting the majority of the world's population, it comes as no surprise that treatment modalities for the reduction of its side effects are always on the rise. Massage therapy is one of the most talked about and researched topics when it comes to benefitting diabetic individuals. In order to better understand as to why this is so, let's take a look at the basic issues that are countered through safe massage techniques for diabetics.

## 1.   The Trigger Points

The overstraining that causes hypersensitivity in a muscle creates trigger points. They are small knots in a muscle formed by contracture of muscle tissue where the blood flow is slow and lacking in nutrients – causing a constant pain, fatigue, and weakness in the muscle. They are also responsible for referral pain.

## 2.   Thickness of blood and thickness of tissue and muscles

To help combat issues related to blood thickness and increased volume of tissue and muscles, massage therapy can be employed. Here, particular movements of the tissues and muscles are stressed upon. This aids to bring about greater flexibility and also eases up muscle and tissue stiffness.

## 3.   Congestion of blood circulation

When it comes to getting a good circulation that's free from the hassle of congestion, massage therapy is the way to go. A full body massage that aims to target the feet and hands region especially is what we are referring to. The full body massage can be carried out either while lying down or more conveniently in the sitting down position. This decision is left up to the client and is based on their feasibility and comfort.

## 4.   Ischemia

This term is taken as the hypersensitivity in soft tissues that is caused by the lack of blood supply. The diabetic Clients are mostly like to have ischemia due to numb muscles.

Now, let's take a look at the massage techniques and how they can benefit from the issues mentioned above in the long run.

### Types of Safe Massage Techniques for Diabetic Individuals

### Diabetic Neuropathy

Diabetic neuropathy is an advanced form of neuromuscular therapy in which specific pressure and deep tissue massage techniques are performed to release the strain in muscle. The technique is applied to the trigger points.

The Art of Massage Aiding in Diabetes, Backache, Anxiety, Depression and Much More

## How Diabetic Neuropathy helps?

So what are the benefits? Well, reduction of blood glucose levels and preventing the neuropathy from getting worse. It can be used to treat soft tissue problems with lower back pain, carpal tunnel symptoms, calf cramps, knee pain, friction syndrome etc.

## Myofascial Release

This specific deep tissue or light tissue massage focuses on the connective muscular tissue. Stiff and snugged connective tissue causes tension in underlying fixtures. Therefore, an adverse effect on posture with severe pain and tension resulted. The myofascial release uses fiber grain technique to stretch the connective tissue and help release posturing fascia of underlying tissue.

## Benefits of MFR

Myofascial Release is highly effective in increasing blood circulation, decreasing pain, posture alignment, and releasing muscular tension. During the sessions, its subtle deep tissue strokes provide relaxation to the diabetic clients and they can experience great relief with toned muscle.

## Shiatsu Massage Therapy

Shiatsu massage is well-known for decreasing pain, nausea, and neuropathy in diabetes. It is a kind of Japanese bodywork that uses fingers, palms, and thumbs to apply on trigger points. The types of shiatsu massage include:

- Hara Shiatsu performed with gentle pressure of breath to release physical and responsive blockages
- Healing Shiatsu is a therapy where the therapist activates the client's own healing potential
- Movement shiatsu is an advanced form of Zen Shiatsu that involves psychotherapy through gestalt principles.

## Benefits of Shiatsu for Diabetic People

This massage therapy is well-known for decreasing stress and anxiety by releasing certain hormones and creating a drop in blood sugar. It also improves blood circulation and insulin absorption in diabetes clients.

## Acu-points for Diabetic Clients

The professional massage therapist understands the certain acu-points to apply acupressure and obtains the beneficial results. To steer clear from an episode of hypoglycemia, the therapists would take special care not to massage over injection areas to prevent absorption of insulin. The pressure points to address in diabetic clients include:

- Liver foot point
- Digestion point
- The back of the knee
- Underneath navel

# CHAPTER 7

# DIABETIC FOOT MASSAGE

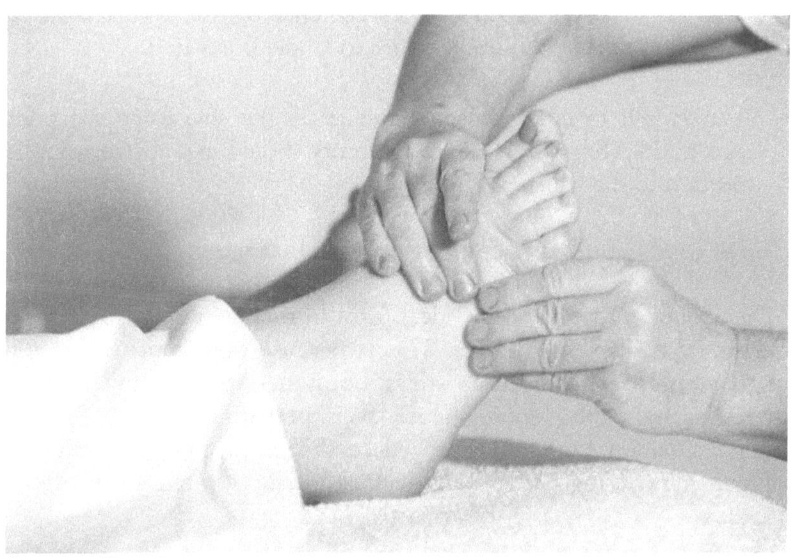

**Source:** Pexels

Feet of a diabetic person are highly affected due to low blood circulation. A good diabetic foot massage can benefit in therapeutic and relaxation forms. It has to be conducted using four simple steps.

- From the heel portion of your foot to the base of your toes, the foot is stroked in a straight line. A back and forth motion is utilized to bring about the greatest effectiveness. The movements are conducted using the heel of the hand or the thumb.

- The toes are wiggled in an outward direction and then pulled in a gentle manner. The area between the toes is massaged using the thumb or the fingers. The next step involves massaging the four metatarsal bones that extend from the top to the middle portion of the foot. The direction to be utilized includes the base of the toes to the area right above the ankle region. Each area must be massaged slowly and with great ease.

- Next, the sole portion of the foot. This area should be given great importance as it is used for carrying the body's weight. The thumb is used to make small circular movements on the sole region. The process is repeated until the entire foot sole is covered.

- Then switch to crosswise movements on the sole using the pointer and middle fingers. These movements should extend from the heel portion to the ball area of the foot.

## Therapeutic Foot Massage

Therapeutic massages are an ideal form of therapy for those individuals suffering from diabetes mellitus. This is because they improve breathing, relax sore muscles and lower stress hormones. Stress only aggravates diabetes as it raises the blood glucose levels, preparing the body for a fight and flight situation. During this procedure, the massage therapist relaxes the body and mind using particular movements that ease tension in the foot muscles.

## Trigger Point Foot Massage

Trigger point therapy is the name given to a type of massage that allows for the application of pressure to certain trigger points of the human body. It is also known as neuromuscular therapy as it affects areas where irritability is present such as knots and lumps the muscle region. The massage allows for the pressure that is acceptable to the diabetic client to be applied to muscles using a number of different movements. This also allows the surrounding muscles to undergo stretching and relaxation. In some clients, this may seem to be a source of discomfort and pain that radiates to

The Art of Massage Aiding in Diabetes, Backache, Anxiety, Depression and Much More

other regions of the body. Trigger point therapy is especially useful in conditions where irregular blood glucose levels lead to muscle cramping in the ankle and calf region due to ischemia.

# CHAPTER 8

## THE SWEDISH THERAPY VS. THE DEEP TISSUE THERAPY

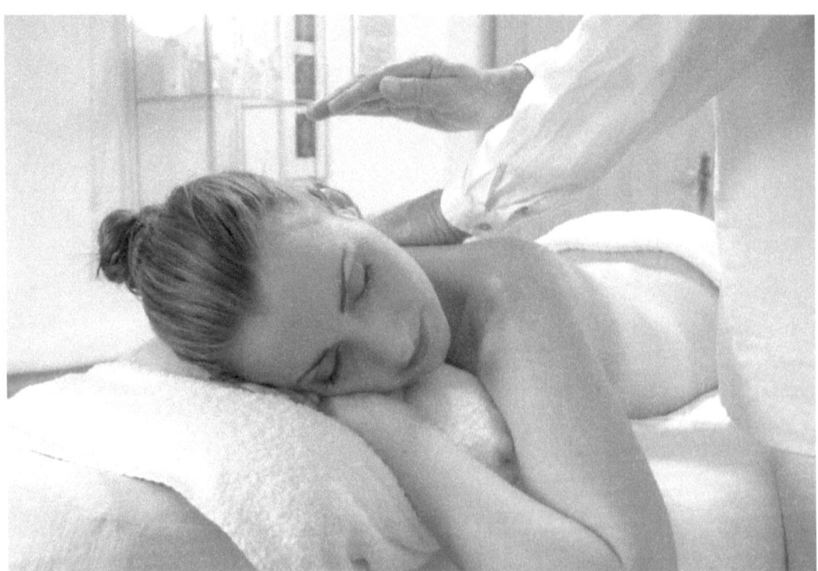

SOURCE: PEXELS

Getting a deep pressure massage is considered as one of the best forms of therapy when it comes to relaxation and soothing of one's senses. Also known as Deep Tissue Massage, but did you know that massage is now considered as a form of therapy used to treat the many side effects of diabetes mellitus? Yes, you heard that right; a massage should never be underestimated, to say the least, because the benefits it can bring are truly fabulous! So what can one expect for the coverage of a healthy and relaxing massage? In order to answer this question, it's essential to view the basics of a Swedish massage and Deep Pressure Massage then go on from there. Also, it doesn't mean that a Deep Tissue Massage will be the best technique for a diabetic especially of the diabetes is not controlled. Therefore, let's take a look.

### What exactly do we mean by the term "Massage Therapy"?

Massage therapy means the manipulation of soft tissue by hand or through a mechanical or electrical apparatus for the purpose of body massage. The term includes effleurage (stroking), petrissage (kneading), tapotement (percussion), compression, vibration, friction, nerve strokes, and Swedish gymnastics. Massage therapy may include the use of oil, lubricant, salt glows, heat lamps, hot and cold packs, or tub, shower, jacuzzi, sauna, steam or cabinet baths. Massage therapy is a healthcare service when the massage is for therapeutic purposes, and a licensed massage therapist may receive referrals from a physician to administer massage therapy. This is the exact definition from TDLR.

A massage can be defined as the act of rubbing the soft tissues of the body. These include the muscles in particular. Massages are great for relieving pain, reducing stress and tension, improving blood flow circulation and promoting the phase of relaxation. There are many different kinds of massages to choose from, each designed in particular for a specific use. Individuals who apply massage are commonly referred to as massage therapists.

A massage therapist may apply pressure using their fingers, hands, elbows and sometimes even shoulders. Massages vary in intensity. Some may be very intense and active, while others are of the milder sort.

### Why Swedish massage techniques differ from others?

Developed by the Swedish doctor Per Henrik Ling, this specific massage has absolutely soothing massage techniques that aid to increase blood circulation, oxygenation, and release toxins like uric acid and lactic acid from the muscles. This is particularly essential for diabetic clients as the build-up of toxins and metabolic waste in their blood is higher due to disturbed pancreatic activity. The Swedish massage also improves muscle flexibility and blood circulation. Let's discuss the different techniques of the classic massage.

### Effleurage

These are gliding and sliding massage methods covering different areas of the body. The therapist gives long sweeping strokes with an alternating light and firm pressure, performed by using fingertips or palm of the hand. For diabetic persons, the pressure is applied according to the case history recommendations.

### Petrissage

This is a prep technique that penetrates deeper massage by kneading of the muscles. It is performed by using various hand techniques to break the pressure points and prepare them for the next massage technique.

### Friction

This technique is the second warm-up set of Swedish massage that prepares the body for deeper pressure point massage. The palms are rubbed together onto the skin of the person being massaged to create a sort of friction. However, this is done on a gentle note in the diabetic clients.

### Rhythmic tapping or Tapotement

The technique involves the sides of the hands' fists that gently taps into a rhythm. This helps in relaxing and energizing the muscles together.

### The Back and Forth Shaking or Vibration

This is done to loosen up the muscles with a heel of the hand in most cases.

### Massage Modalities

There are a number of different types of massages that take place. The type varies on the need or want of the client. Some common types of massages include the following:

- Trigger point massage
- Sports massage
- Swedish massage
- Self-massage

The Art of Massage Aiding in Diabetes, Backache, Anxiety, Depression and Much More

**Trigger point massage-** the name of this massage is self-explanatory for its description. It is a form of massage that focuses on particular trigger points located in various regions throughout the body. It is a less gentle form of massage, considered as uncomfortable to many. Pressure is applied by the massage therapist to various regions of the body such as knots, muscle ties, and tense/overworked muscles. The massage is carried out till the muscles are at complete ease.

**Sports massage-** deep tissue massage is another form of massage that is of the active and tense sort. The long-lasting tension of the muscles can usually be treated by this form of massage. Slow strokes are applied by the massage therapist using the elbows and fingers. This is done with the effort of reaching the deeper layers of the muscle region. As a diabetic, it is recommended doing brisk walking at 30 minutes a day. This from time to time may aggravate the joints and posture, and a light sports massage will aid with pain, posture, and elasticity.

**Swedish massage-** one of the most gentle and soft therapies. This type of massage uses a number of different techniques used to promote muscle tension relief, improvement in blood circulation and greater relaxation. Techniques commonly employed in this type of massage include gliding strokes, tapping and kneading methods on the muscle layer that is in the direction of the heart's blood flow.

When it comes to a good massage, it is undoubtedly a useful form of treatment. We'll discuss as to why this may be the case. Firstly, massages promote relaxation like none other. Other than that, a massage is able to relieve pain in a way that's convenient, cost-effective and doesn't require medical intervention.

Massages are considered as a great form of therapy to relieve different kinds of muscle tension. Blood flow restoration and enhancement of circulation of blood around the body are also some great benefits that massages possess. Pain resulting due to pressure on the nerves is another ailment that clients can relieve through the usage of a massage. Lastly, lost joint movement can be restored like never before.

## What precautions should be taken to ensure that your massage is totally safe?

When it comes to massage therapy, few risks are generally associated with the procedure overall. This is provided for the fact that a trained professional is undertaking the massage. Going into a massage, one should feel totally relaxed. There are however a number of precautions that should be taken so as to avoid any sort of mishap during the procedure. The following conditions are such that they require consultation with the doctor before a massage can be implemented.

These include the following:

1.  Open wound areas
2.  Areas of weak skin
3.  Veins possessing blood clots
4.  Bruises
5.  Known bleeding disorder
6.  Drug history that involves usage of a blood thinner
7.  A general overall decrease of blood platelet counts
8.  Pregnant women should avoid taking a massage. If your health care provider is ok with it, then only should massages be availed during pregnancy.
9.  Clients suffering from a tumor or cancer should avoid the application of deep as well as intense pressure on the skin surface where the tumor or cancer is present. Again, this should be approved by the client's health care provider.

## What is a good Deep Tissue Massage?

We've usually come across the term good massage. With that being said, however, not many people out there are actually aware of what a good massage actually entails. A good massage is a term given to a massage that utilizes a healing touch for the reduction of heart rate, stress levels, hormones in the blood and blood pressure. Other than that, a good massage will work to enhance the body's immune function. It can act to also raise the levels of the body's natural painkillers which are known as endorphins and serotonin too.

Good massages also influence the rate of mood regulators release, all at the expense of relieving soreness of achy muscles. The best advice I may give is that if that massage shouldn't be painful. If you in pain and you

The Art of Massage Aiding in Diabetes, Backache, Anxiety, Depression and Much More

cannot tolerate it, then make your therapist aware. Unless you are challenging your body to have more elasticity or range of motion you bet there will be discomfort, but never do more than you can tolerate. Listen to your body! This is the big advice for you today!

## LISTEN TO YOUR BODY!

# CHAPTER 9

## STRESS MANAGEMENT / RELAXATION THROUGH DIABETIC MASSAGE TECHNIQUES

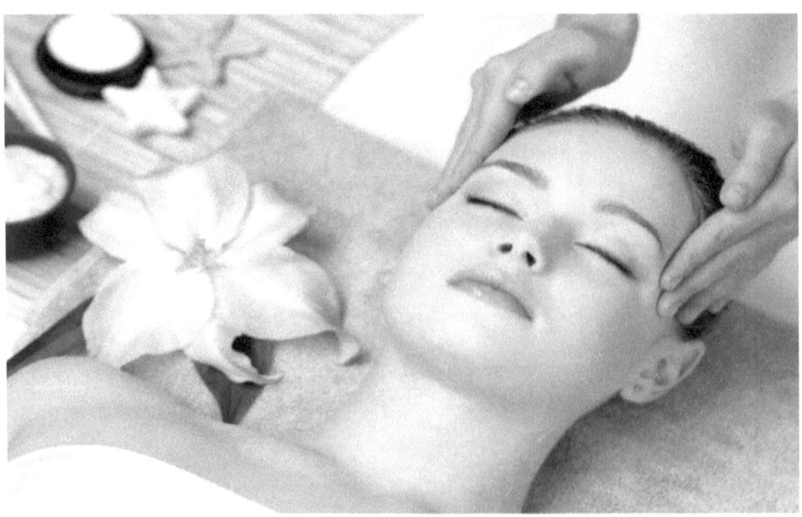

Source: 123RF

With all the hustle and bustle of this world, it's hard for normal individuals to let alone diabetics to manage stress in today's day and age. Massages are considered a great form of therapy with numerous benefits being mentioned previously. Techniques for relaxation are an essential aspect of the management of stress. Stress is known to take a toll on one's mind, body, and soul. For this reason, researchers are always on the lookout for methods through which stress can be tackled. There are a number of ways through which an individual can cope with stress, allowing your mind

The Art of Massage Aiding in Diabetes, Backache, Anxiety, Depression and Much More

to focus on greater attention and help lower your rate of breathing.

## How to go about coping with stress?

With the rate at which the world moves and the challenges that everyday life brings, coping with stress has never been so important. There are a number of ways through which you can go about handling stress.

- **Step 1- Identify triggers to monitor what it actually is that stresses you out.**

This can range from things as basic choices as what food should I consume today, and weather conditions to more complex situations such as medical conditions, relationships, personal traumas, emotions, work. Watch for this particular in diabetes mellitus.

- **Step 2- Think of ways or strategies on how you plan on dealing with stress.**

This strategy can involve a whole array of things. Seeking professional help, outdoor activities such as sports or simply talking to yourself to let those emotions out.

### Massaging your brain –the ideal method for stress relief

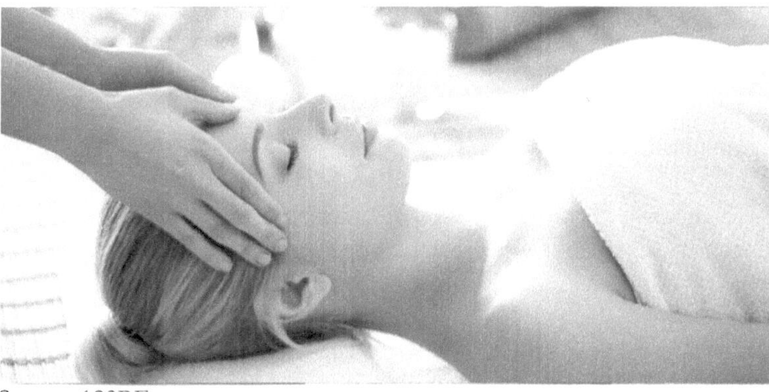

Source: 123RF

Massages are a wonderful form of therapy when it comes to relief from stress and the ultimate mode of relaxation. The end result we may add is a general sense of well-being.

## Stress is all in your head

To help understand why it is that massages bring about a general decrease in stress, one should be well aware of the neurotransmitters and hormones that control a person's moods.

- **Serotonin**

It is the name given to a specialized hormone secreted in the brain that regulates mood, amongst other things like hunger and sleep. During a massage, serotonin is promoted to be released by the brain. This is why a positive mood usually is observed after an individual undergoes a massage.

- **Dopamine**

It is the name given to a neurotransmitter whose levels increase after a massage. The neurons that are attached to dopamine are the same as those responsible for providing a sense of reward system. Feelings of well-being, pleasure, and content are some of the many emotions attached to this neurotransmitter.

- **Oxytocin**

It is the name given to the hormone of love as it provides a feeling of warmth, fading away with time. During a massage, this hormone is elevated to high levels, especially when the massage is of the gentle or mild type. It is this hormone that gives one that feeling of care and comfort, similar to that being treated in a spa.

- **Cortisol**

Cortisol is a hormone released into the body when stress levels are at an ultimate high, which is why it's renowned as the stress hormone. It constricts blood vessels, causing blood pressure to increase.

During a massage, the levels of cortisol are found to drastically decrease. As a result of this, the physiological effects of stress are automatically lowered too. This simultaneously also increases the body's immunity to viruses and improves healing of wounds.

The Art of Massage Aiding in Diabetes, Backache, Anxiety, Depression and Much More

- **Epinephrine or Nor-epinephrine/ Adrenaline or Nor-adrenaline**

These hormones are the ones responsible for the body's fight or flight reaction, which in turn is directly linked to stress.

During a massage, the levels of these hormones are dramatically decreased to an ultimate low. To summarize, all the feelings related to a sense of relaxation is what you can expect. Some of the common effects observed in the human body after a massage due to their decrease include.

- ✓ Increased glucose metabolism
- ✓ Lowered blood pressure
- ✓ Lowered heart rate

## Evidence related to massages causing an ultimate sense of well-being and relaxation

According to a study released by the Touch Research Institute, massages have been found to create a long-lasting effect on the brain like no other form of stress relief. Massages help to increase delta waves. These waves are necessarily linked to deep sleep. One of the main reasons why individuals tend to fall asleep on the massage table is related to this phenomenon. To simply put it, a massage tends to shift the balance away from all modes of everyday stress and tilts it towards feelings of well-being, motivation, relaxation, and healing. What more can one ask for?

## Diabetic Clients can now get the relaxation they need through a Neural Massage

Living and overcoming the many challenges associated with diabetes mellitus carries with it a bundle of stress. The value of living a stress-free life can never be underestimated. The body's systems are on a constant strain at the majority of the time when blood sugar levels are high. Other than that, worrying about the complications of the disease as well as the anxiety related to work or everyday relationships can add to your pile of stress.

Massages can help calm the nervous system down. Other than that, a massage works to bring about rest to the mind and body. This is all known to have a profound effect on the body's inner chemical balance, helping to rid the body of stress hormones. All it takes is to skillfully apply touch to the right areas and you can soon wave stress related to diabetes goodbye.

# CHAPTER 10

## MASSAGE TIPS AND PRECAUTIONS FOR DIABETIC CLIENTS

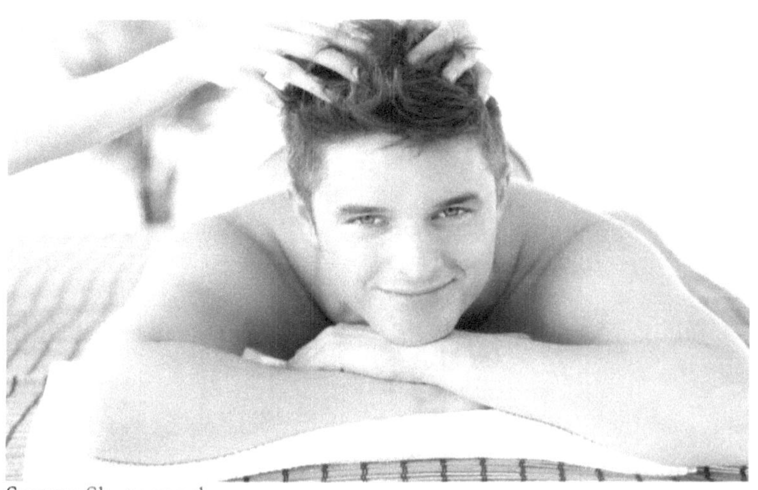

Source: Shutterstock

Diabetes Mellitus is prevalent amongst a majority; therefore, naturally, various treatments have been put to the test to either serve as an alternative to Western medicine or to simply aid Western medicine in the recovery process. Herbal medicine is one of those alternatives that have found significant recognition especially amongst the population that conforms to the taboos associated with the extensive use of Western medicine.

Although initially put under a lot of fire for not being effective or practical enough, herbal medicine has proved to be a surefire way of controlling diabetes. Similarly, massage therapy has been the subject of widespread speculation but multiple types of research carried out over the years now confidently vouch for the effect of this primitive seemingly ineffective technique. While it is not of much benefit to the client when implemented on its own but when used in conjunction with an alternative mode of treatment, it can reap promising results. People who employed massage therapy showed more progress towards betterment compared to those who only stuck with medicine for diabetic monitoring.

Just like any other mode of treatment, this one too comes with its own set of repercussions. Awareness can only be achieved by actively involving one's self into research and study revolving around certain topics. When it comes to your body and treatment for ailments, one who is unaware of the complexities associated with each and every body part must restrain themselves from taking any major treatment decisions derived solely from their own judgment. Therefore, it is wise to consult your doctor beforehand and discuss each and every detail with them. Your consulting professional will guide you regarding any unfortunate outcomes of the treatment if any and also give you the best advice based on your condition.

Similarly, all health care professionals must be well aware of the expectations, repercussions, and outcomes associated with the treatment method they are offering. Physical therapy healthcare providers are just as crucial to the healthcare sector as any other healthcare provider. When it comes to massage therapists, there are certain things one must know especially when dealing with a client with Diabetes Mellitus.

## 10 Important Factors Diabetic Clients Must Consider while Going for Message Therapy

Similarly, for a client, if he or she is considering opting for massage therapy, they should be well equipped with all possible information regarding the treatment. Following are some tips that will help every diabetic client should employ in order to reap maximum benefits.

### Make sure to do a background check with your therapist regarding your condition.

It is important to be open with your therapist when undergoing the process of seeking massage. A detailed and thorough history forms the basis of any future therapy; therefore, do not hesitate in front of your therapist when explaining your condition. Talk about every minute detail associated with your condition to ensure a secure therapist-client

The Art of Massage Aiding in Diabetes, Backache, Anxiety, Depression and Much More

relationship and also the best possible massage results.

### Be honest about any progress.

Feedback is crucial in order to determine progress. If you feel a significant improvement in your condition, let your therapist know. If you feel like you are still standing where you started, let your therapist know. Your feedback will enable your health care provider to make the necessary modifications required if they are to strive towards betterment. Be open with your health care provider and you will notice significant changes.

### Do not be afraid to voice your fears or your concerns.

If there is anyone who can push away your fears and concerns, it is your health care provider. Discuss your concerns with them before you sign any forms. Only if you are convinced should you go ahead with the treatment otherwise you have the right to terminate treatment at any given point. Your therapist knows best regarding the complications and negative outcomes that may be associated with something. Talk to them without any hesitation.

### Discuss breaks with your therapist.

Feeling too overwhelmed and desperately craving a break? Talk to your therapist. All treatments require consistency and often times the routine gets quite hectic and exhausting. If you are looking for a break, do not beat yourself up. Let your therapist know how you have been feeling. Taking a leave of absence without informing your health care provider not only disrupts the routine but it also hinders the treatment process that does more harm than good.

### Harbor realistic expectations.

Like any supplementary treatment, massage therapy is not a miracle worker. You cannot expect it to heal you completely without making any other individual efforts such as diet and portion control and regular exercise. We as clients tend to set unrealistic expectations when it comes to treatment. Start off with a realistic goal. Discuss any thoughts you might be having with your therapist before you start treatment in order to avoid disappointment later.

## Consult your physician first.

The most important factor is to consult your doctor before you set an appointment with a therapist. Listen to your doctor's advice. Only proceed if your doctor green lights your proposition. If they advise you against it, best steer clear of it because, in the end, a doctor knows best.

## Keep a regular check of your blood glucose levels.

Check and balance is what will ensure progress. Regularly monitor your blood sugar levels using strip tests and maintain a record. Recovery patterns are what will determine your progress and hence the effectiveness of the employed treatment. It's crucial to check your sugar levels at least 4 times in a day so as to determine whether or not the massage can benefit. In situations where you're not feeling well, sugar levels should be checked more frequently.

## Always perform the massage in an air-conditioned room when temperatures reach an absolute high

During the summertime when temperatures reach 85 degrees and above, it's important to perform activities like massages indoors. Being diabetic, sweating and dehydration are an absolute no and are considered as dangerous.

Stay hydrated at all times. To avoid any unfortunate circumstance during the massage, drink plenty of water at all times. This helps to keep you hydrated and avoids fainting spells.

Keep a lookout for signals that may indicate heat exhaustion or lowering of blood glucose levels

There is a list of symptoms to keep a lookout for when undertaking a massage. These include the following:
- Fainting
- Dizziness
- Excessive sweating
- Cramps in the muscles
- Raised heartbeat rate
- Feeling of nausea
- Vomiting

- Appearance of cool and clammy skin
- Sudden rise of headaches
- Personality change
- Pounding of the heart
- Inability to waken
- Change in personality
- Impaired vision
- Shaking and trembling

If any of the above symptoms arise, it's best to inform the massage therapist to stop the procedure until conditions return to absolutely normal. This is because these are all symptoms of hypoglycemia or low blood sugar and can be considered fatal. The massage therapist must know how to deal with the situation in a professional manner. In cases where an emergency arises, an immediate call for professional medical help should be sought.

Individuals diagnosed with type 2 diabetes or non-insulin dependent diabetes are those who do not depend on insulin to treat their elevated blood sugar levels. Proper diet, lifestyle modifications, and care are required for these types of clients. When it comes to massages, there are a number of precautions that must be administered when treating type 2 diabetic clients. If effectively followed, these clients can safely enjoy the many benefits that entail massage therapy. These include improvement in blood glucose levels, control of stress levels, a decrease in blood pressure and avoidance of long-term complications such as a diabetic foot.

While massage therapy is excellent in terms of physical as well as psychological healing, there are other measures that must be taken in order to reap the best results. Switch to a healthier diet, regular exercise, and make smarter life choices in addition to seeking any kind of therapy. Follow these diligently and we guarantee positive results.

# CHAPTER 11

# IMPORTANT ADVICE TO MASSAGE THERAPISTS AND CLIENTS

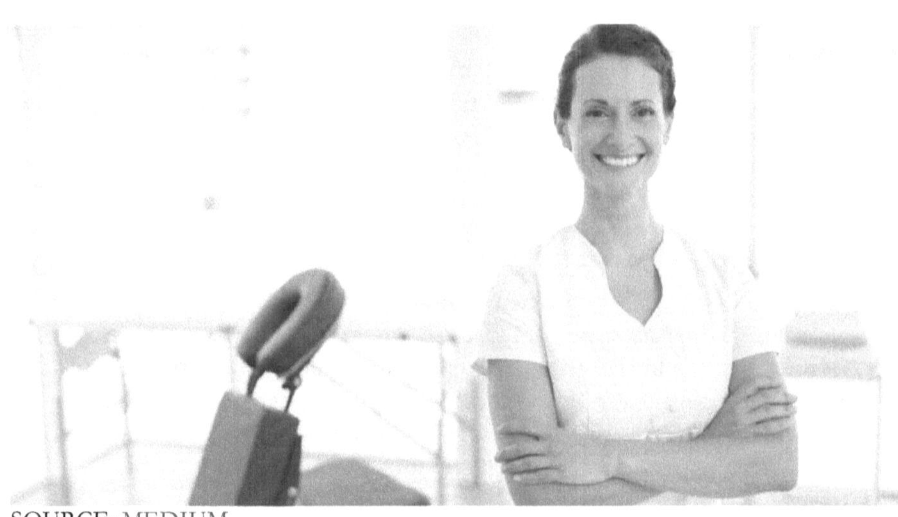

SOURCE: MEDIUM

Being a diabetic and going for a massage requires special care and attention. Having awareness of the client's condition and how to attend to their desired needs and requirements is so important. Other than that, having thorough knowledge about how to deal with an emergency condition that revolves around hypoglycemia is crucial. With the following advice being mentioned below, massage therapists can expect to provide the most promising and long-lasting effects of the massage therapy to their

The Art of Massage Aiding in Diabetes, Backache, Anxiety, Depression and Much More

diabetic clients.

## Be well aware of the precautions associated with treating a diabetic client

Systemic diseases such as Diabetes Mellitus must be handled with the utmost care. When treating a diabetic client, be sure to accustom yourself to the necessary information about the condition. This includes signs, symptoms, complications, and most importantly, precautions. Before proceeding with any kind of treatment, take a detailed history of the client's condition. The more detailed your background check; the better the outcome will be.

## Always put into practical implementation the technique whose complications you are aware of.

We as human beings are not perfect. We are not programmed to know anything and everything. When dealing with a diabetic client or any client in general, do not practically implement any technique that you even remotely unsure of. Only go ahead with the ones you are good at and know everything about.

## Be very careful when employing pressure techniques as they may contribute to worsening the client's condition.

The human body comprises of multiple pressure points; each serving their own purpose in physiological functioning. Needless to say, pressure point techniques should be practiced with utmost care in order to avoid any mishaps.

You should be aware of rapid fluctuations of glucose levels in the blood during the therapy session. During a massage, the body is in a state of peace and relaxation. For this reason, they may not be able to sense a change that occurs in their body at that particular moment in time. Having vast knowledge about hypoglycemia and its symptoms is necessary. Other than that, being alert about the symptoms of changes in blood glucose levels in your client is necessary at that particular point in time

### Know the core techniques involved in treating a diabetic client.

Specific conditions should be dealt with in a specific mannerism. Some techniques that are commonly employed for diabetic individuals include Lymph drainage massage, Swedish style massage, Deep tissue therapy, Shiatsu-style massage, Therapeutic touch massage and Comfort Touch Massage. Each client varies in type and condition. Studying the client's condition from beforehand and then attempting the particular style is particularly useful. It is prudent to ensure that you employ therapies according to specific needs of your individual client.

### Always listen to the client's feedback.

Feedback is crucial if you need to record the client's condition's betterment. Be open and accepting and allow the client to garner their trust in you. This helps invoke a strong sense of security in the client as well. If the client complains of any form of pain or discomfort during the massage therapy, the session should be stopped and modifications may be attempted. Never should a particular technique be enforced upon a client. After listening to a client's feedback and views about the massage therapy session, modifications in the massage style may be attempted.

If you wish to become a successful massage therapist, be open and receptive to any sort of feedback being communicated your way. This entails encouraging the diabetic client to share information with you about their condition and personal care.

Feedback carries great value when it comes to a massage. Every client should be given great priority and this can be done by listening to feedback. Any form of constructive criticism should be worked upon so as to make the therapy a rewarding one for the client. In short, listening to the client is key.

### If there are any changes you would like to make, always take your client's consent.

It is wise to always inform the client regarding any changes that you would like to introduce in the therapy routine. The core teachings of medicine stress the importance of having the client's consent before proceeding with any procedure; even something as minute as asking them what their presenting complaint is. This protocol is no different. Let your client know every detail.

The Art of Massage Aiding in Diabetes, Backache, Anxiety, Depression and Much More

### Never push your client into engaging in something they are not fully comfortable with.

If you feel like a certain technique could bring more benefit to the client, let them know. If the client seems hesitant, do not push them or insist them into doing something they are not 100% comfortable with.

### Build a trustworthy bond with your client.

Instigate healthy relations with your clients. Be open to questions of all sorts and express your concern. The therapist-client relationship is a very sacred bond. Allow your client to feel at ease when in your presence. This will ensure honest conversation and thus the best treatment outcome.

### Know the physical symptoms associated with decreased blood glucose levels.

Massage therapy is renowned for being very relaxing. The major warning that comes with diabetes is fluctuating glucose levels. Often times, blood glucose levels can fall quite low mid-treatment. While the client may be unable to process it soon, it is your duty to pick up on any evident physical signs associated with fluctuating glucose levels. Take the necessary measures to ensure no episodes of hypoglycemia or subsequent fainting ensue.

### Study Your Client History

Before undertaking a particular style of massage upon a diabetic client, the complications of the condition must be thoroughly studied. Never blindly attempt a style as it may result in dire consequences.

### Be Sure About What Massage Technique has to be applied

Pressure should never be applied in excessive amounts. Techniques that involve the use of pressure should be administered within acceptable limits and under the knowledge of the client. Styles that the therapist is doubtful about may make matters worse.

## Keep it Gentle

Aggression is a trait that can ruin many phenomena. Massage therapy works best when handled with care. A soft touch brings more benefit than a rough one. Adopting a lighter approach with a gentle touch is the best way to go about dealing with diabetic clients. This way, you're bound to be on the safer side in most conditions.

## Give Awareness to your client

Discuss the physical and psychological benefits of massage therapy for diabetic clients. This makes clients look forward to their massage therapy with greater vigor. Also be willing to guide them on how they can make the results of this therapy session last longer with maintaining a balanced diet, proper exercise, and lifestyle modifications. A little thought can go a long way when it comes to therapy and counseling.

The Art of Massage Aiding in Diabetes, Backache, Anxiety, Depression and Much More

# CONCLUSION

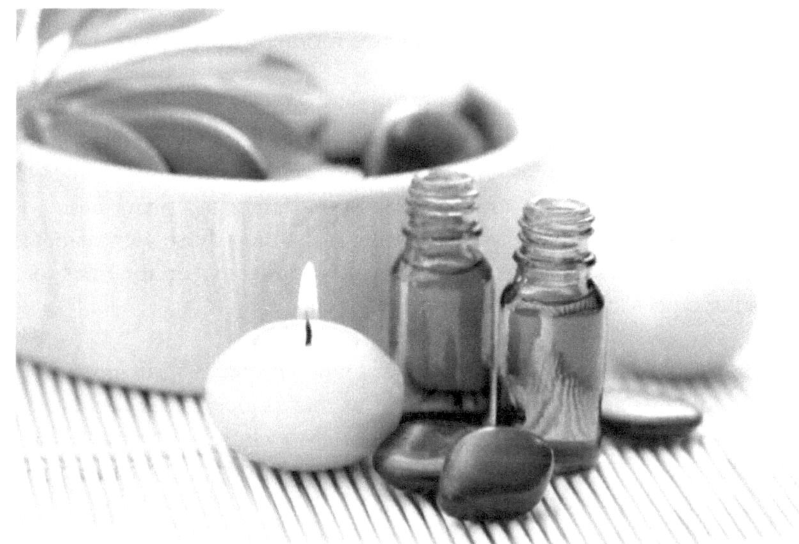

Diabetes mellitus is the name given to a medical condition where impaired glucose metabolism takes place. This means the body is unable to adequately store and make use of glucose in the body. A common finding is high levels of glucose in the blood at all times.

 This glucose is most commonly excreted out in the urine which is why frequent urination (polyuria) and frequent thirst (polydipsia) are commonly observed.

Diabetes mellitus can be of two types, where type 1 is concerned with lack of insulin being produced by the body's pancreas and type 2 is related to lack of sensitivity of the body's target receptors to the hormone that controls glucose uptake, insulin.

The complications related to diabetes mellitus are comprehensive, ranging from simple to moderate and then severe. Diabetic retinopathy affects the eyes whereas diabetic neuropathy affects the digestive tract and peripheries, especially the legs and feet. The microvasculature and circulatory system is also affected, alongside damage and thickening of the muscles and fascia. Heart disease is common in diabetic clients and so is damage to the kidneys and urinary bladder. The skin may undergo multiple infections, especially in the calf region. In severe circumstances, gangrene may lead to foot or complete leg amputation.

Treating diabetes is a lifelong struggle for those involved in the condition. Careful thought, planning, diet control, lifestyle modifications and personal care encompass a long-lasting and effective mode of treatment.

Medical intervention is of greatest importance when it comes to treatment for diabetes mellitus. With that being said, however, coping with the side effects and stress that comes with the baggage of diabetes is sometimes too much to handle for anyone out there. Massage therapy is a proved and effective treatment modality when it comes to helping those with diabetes mellitus. Professional massage therapy works wonders when it comes to benefitting type 1 and type 2 diabetic individuals.

What makes massage therapy so beneficial when it comes to treating diabetic individuals is a question many of us may ponder upon. Believe it or not, the answer is simple. All it takes is the right technique, the right type of touch and the proper area to which the massage is administered.

Some of the most common forms of massage techniques and styles used for diabetic individuals involve Swedish massage, Trigger point therapy, deep therapeutic massage and Sports massage. It's all about employing the right amount of pressure and correct technique, and it won't be too long to feel the difference.

Massage therapy does not bring with it any side effects. Some of the known benefits include helping to improve the body's congested blood circulation, increased mobility, reduction of stress hormones in the debilitated client, greater tissue elasticity, improved intake of the cells' to insulin and a general sense of relaxation and wellbeing amongst all others.

A person's physical and mental health is the greatest gift one can possibly possess in an era where diseases and ailments are at an all-time high. With massage therapy, individuals can find an immediate sense of relief that

The Art of Massage Aiding in Diabetes, Backache, Anxiety, Depression and Much More

encompasses deep restful relaxation while helping to reduce the many complications of their diabetic condition.

Quick Tips to be followed by type 2 diabetic Clients when undertaking a massage:

•      Every diabetic client should inform their massage therapist of their particular condition and needs to be fulfilled.

•      Feedback is so crucial when getting a massage. Being honest and displaying feedback is the best way to go about the situation. This will ensure the current massage experience and the next one to come will be a pleasurable one.

•      Any comments and queries should be dealt with before the procedure begins. This is done to ensure that no doubt is left in the mind of the client upon whom the massage is done. Only when the mind is stress and doubts free can the massage be termed beneficial.
•      If a break is desired during the massage, it should be availed at all costs. Many individuals may find a massage a new experience and so dealing with it may be overwhelming for some.

•      Never go into a massage expecting wonders to take place. Massage alongside a good balanced diet and performance of regular exercises is so important for the best results.

•      Keeping a regular check on the blood glucose levels is important as it is the best indicator of the effects of the therapy undertaken. Other than that, it's also important to know how much improvement you can expect to achieve through massage therapy. Having unnecessarily high blood sugar levels will lead to little or no improvement from massage therapy.

•      Before undertaking a massage, it's important to arrange a consultation with your medical doctor. Once you get the green signal to go ahead, the massage can be enjoyed with greater pleasure.

# ABOUT THE AUTHOR

I am a Professional Massage Therapist with over ten years of experience, and with over six years of experience teaching theory and practice of therapeutic massage. Now, I am also dedicated to Professional Massage, Diabetes, & Weight-loss awareness.

I obtained professional training in multiple massage therapy modalities including Active Release Techniques, Deep Tissue Therapy, Sports Massage, Myofascial Release, Injury Rehabilitation, Swedish massage, and basic Neurokinetic Therapy.

I taught Massage Therapy Principles for six years at a college in Texas. During my teaching period at Western Technical College, I was able to meet many people, and exchange many experiences, but the most challenging experience for me was the following:

I was diagnosed with diabetes at the age of thirty. Along with the medical treatment, exercise, and diet, I aided myself with the knowledge of massage therapy and got outstanding results. I believe that with the right kind of technique, massage can work wonders in diabetes and other medical conditions.

 I also went from being 240 lbs. – 140 lbs. I had to learn the hard way! On the other hand, it opened my eyes. I understood how much I was harming my body. Therefore, I opted to make changes. I understand it's difficult to keep a positive attitude in times of devastation, but I have a new plan now! I want to make others aware of the wonders of Massage Therapy in Diabetes, Anxiety, Depression, Cancer, Arthritis, Stress and much more.

This book emphasizes its content on massage and Diabetes Mellitus. If you are a Massage Therapist this book may be useful as a quick reference. If you are in the medical field you might find this book elemental, but it is about awareness.

I hope you enjoyed this book & Thank you for your time and purchase.

Love,
Brenda